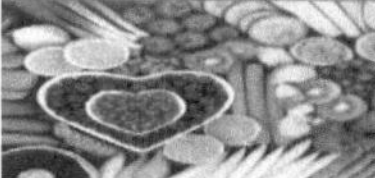

Contents

Title	page number
The food pyramid	1
Carbohydrates	2
Proteins	2
Fats	3
water	4
Vitamins	4
Folic acid	6
Calcium	6
Iron	6
Zinc	7
The needs of pregnant and breastfeeding women	8
Dietary advice for a pregnant woman	12
Dietary advice for a nursing mother	13
Breastfeeding	13
The benefits of breastfeeding	15
Correct breastfeeding	16
Working breastfeeding mother	18
The risks of artificial feeding on a child	19
Complementary foods and breastfeeding	20
Rules for introducing complementary feeding	20
Improve adolescent nutrition	26
personal cleanliness	27
House cleanliness	29

The food pyramid

Sugar

Proteins, cheese and milk

carbohydrate

Fruits and Vegetables

Liquids, Water and Juices

Carbohydrates:

It is divided into three sections:

Monosaccharide's:

Like sugar, candy, most biscuits, ready-made sponge cake, and it is digested and absorbed into the body faster than other sugars

Dual sugars:

Like the sugar in milk

Compound sugars:

Like potatoes, flour, whole grains, such as:

Rice and pasta are the best sugars that stay in your body for a long time

Importance:

An energy source for the whole body, and in particular it benefits the nervous system (the brain) as a basic and fast food that helps to get rid of waste regularly, as well as building body cells

Proteins:

It is divided into two parts:

Animal source: **includes red meat, fish, liver, eggs and white meat**

Plant source: **grains and legumes, such as: lentils, beans, and beans**

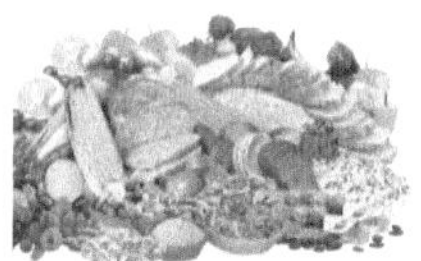

Carbohydrates

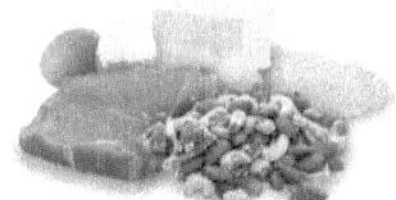

Proteins

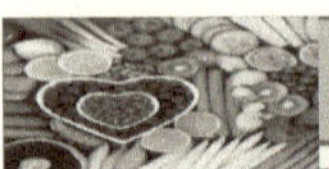

Importance:

An energy source, important for building cells and making up for damage from them. It enters the body's cells, such as muscles and blood, fighting infections.

The daily requirement is every 1 kg of the human body needs 1 g of protein, for example: a child weighing 13 kg needs 13 g of protein, i.e. (1 g of protein gives 4 calories)

Fats:

It is divided into two parts:

Saturated fats: they are solid or liquid fats that are converted to solid (i.e. hydrogenation process), such as: cream, butter, animal fats, obesity.

Unsaturated fats: they are plant-based liquid fats, such as: olive oil, sunflower oil, corn oil

Importance:

Fat is a source of energy, it enters the structure of body cells, regulates the body's processes by supplying it with fat-soluble vitamins (every 1 g of fat gives 4 calories).

Note:

Eating saturated fats causes obesity and atherosclerosis, preferably by replacing it with unsaturated fats.

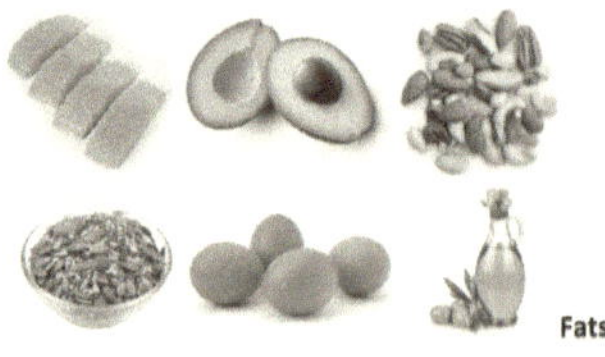

Fats

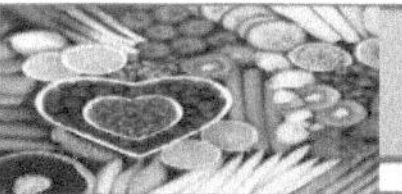

water:

Each person needs to drink 2 to 3 liters of water per day (approximately 8 to 10 cups of 250 mm)

Importance:

Maintains body temperature, maintains blood volume as a mean of transporting nutrients, prevents dehydration, enters metabolic processes such as digesting carbohydrates, starches, proteins, fats

Vitamins:

It is divided into two parts:

Fat-soluble vitamins:

Vitamin A: found in colored vegetables such as: carrots, cabbage, pumpkins, apricots, sweet potatoes, and also found in the liver, kidneys, brain, butter

Its importance:

Maintains eye tissue, protects against night blindness, protects the skin and its components (called: beauty vitamins) and strengthens immunity

Vitamin D:

It is found in sardines, salmon, tuna, eggs, cheese and butter, and the UV rays of the sun are also activated upon exposure to the formation of vitamin D subcutaneous

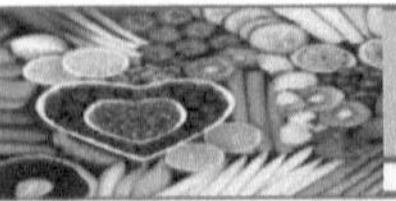

Its importance:

Prevents bone softening in children, prevents osteoporosis in adults, stimulates the immune system and strengthens the work of the central nervous system

Vitamin E:

It is found in vegetable oils, nuts, avocados, and liver

Its importance:

Activates skin immunity, lining of the respiratory tract and mucous membranes, contributes to the production of red blood cells, improves fertilization rates

Vitamin K:

It is found in dark-colored vegetables, such as spinach, hibiscus, and chives

Its importance:

Prevents bleeding, helps blood clotting

Water soluble vitamins are: **B2, B2, B2, B2, B2, folic acid, vitamin C:**

Vitamin B1 is necessary for growth and functioning of the nervous system

Food sources rich in vitamin B are: liver, meat, sardines, cabbage, spinach, avocado, whole grains, dairy products, .bananas, yeast

Its importance:

It contributes to the synthesis of brain and nerve cells, enters the synthesis of red blood cells, strengthens immunity

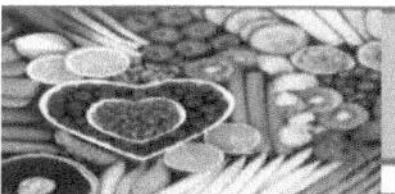

vitamin C:

It is found in (lemon, orange, guava, kiwi, green pepper)

Its importance:

Helps absorb iron, helps skin freshness, helps heal wounds and prevent bleeding

Folic acid:

It is found in dark and colored leafy vegetables as well as in peas, oranges, and dairy

Its importance:

Prevents fetal deformity, strengthens the nervous system, prevents some types of anemia

Calcium:

It is found in (dairy, cheese, sardines, white sesame)

Its importance:

It includes bone and teeth structure, helps blood to clot. The child needs daily (270-400 mg daily).

Iron:

There are two sources:

Animal source: **meat, fish, eggs, liver**

Plant source: **lentils, beans, peas, dried fruits, dark green leafy vegetables, such as: mallow, hibiscus, spinach**

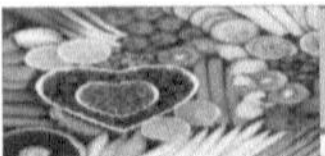

It is included in the structure of red blood cells, preventing anemia

Zinc:

found in (red meat, peanuts, sunflower oil, whole grains)

Its importance:

It helps to grow and prevents stunting

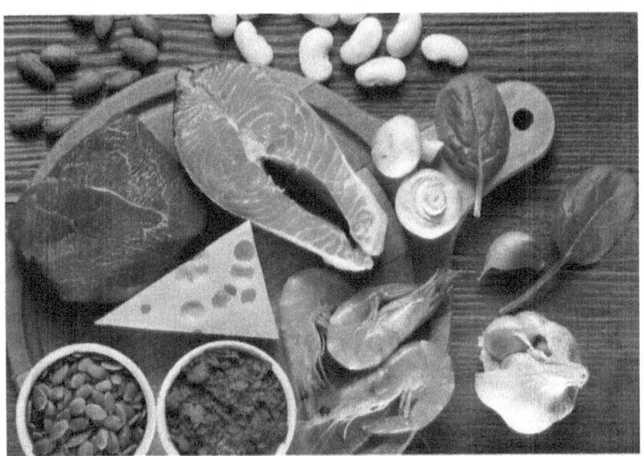

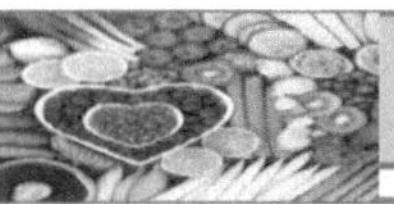

The mother's interest in her health and nutrition before and during pregnancy is necessary for her health and her ability to bear children, especially since the reproductive period puts the mother under the need for complete and balanced nutrition to cover many important physiological functions, as well as for the formation and growth of the fetus and for the formation of new tissues during pregnancy, and for the formation of the necessary milk during breastfeeding.

Nutrient and pregnant needs of nutrients:

The pregnant and breastfeeding needs of energy and nutrients increase in order to cover many important physiological functions at this stage. Among the most important needs are:

Energy: **Energy requirements increase by (300 kilocalories / day) during pregnancy and by (500 kilocalories per day) for breastfeeding women**

Protein: **The daily requirements of the protein for the breastfeeder increase at a rate of (15 g), and the pregnant woman needs additional quantities at the rate of (10 g), and the most important food sources rich in protein (meat, poultry, fish and eggs, dairy products, legumes, nuts and nuts)**

Vitamins: Vitamin A:

It is recommended to increase vitamin A during pregnancy by eating rich sources such as leafy vegetables and yellow colored fruits (carrots, apricots, melons), liver and kidneys. It is recommended to increase vitamin A during the breastfeeding

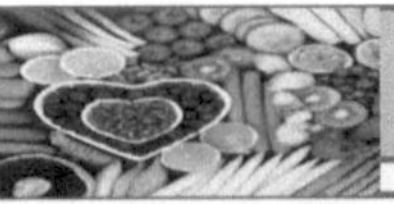

It is advised to increase the vitamin C for a pregnant woman, as the importance of this vitamin lies in the formation of the collagen (collagen) during the active division of cells in the stage of fetal development. Sources of vitamin C fruits, fresh citrus fruits such as: green pepper and guava.

Folic acid:

The importance of this vitamin comes due to its importance in cell division, which makes the need of the fetus great for it, and it is perhaps one of the most important problems of nutritional deficiency during pregnancy, and therefore it is given as additional doses for pregnant women who have anemia or even as a prevention from the occurrence of this type of anemia, and the most important Sources: Tomato juice, avocado, sunflower seeds, leafy vegetables, lentils and citrus.

For mineral elements:

The need for all nutrients increases during pregnancy and for breastfeeding, to become at its peak during the third trimester of pregnancy, as pregnant women need calcium found in white sesame, dairy products, iron found in red meat, liver, green leafy vegetables and legumes to cover the fetus's need.

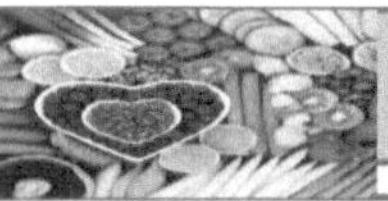

Nutrition accompanying a pregnant woman's troubles:

Pregnant women may experience some of the troubles of the first pregnancy, especially in the early hours of the day, and it may extend to the rest of the day accompanied by vomiting sometimes, and this may be due to disturbances in hormonal secretions at the beginning of pregnancy, and to alleviate these problems the following can be followed:

.Drink liquids between meals and not with them, especially in the early morning

.Avoid fatty fried foods and spices

.Eat slowly with good chewing

Increase the number of meals while reducing the amount of food per .serving

Increased intake of fiber-rich foods such as whole grains, fruits, .vegetables and legumes

.Do some exercise

Dietary guidelines for a pregnant mother:

.Eat a balanced diet and stay away from bad eating habits

.Food diversification

.Maintaining the natural increase in weight

.(Moderation in stimulants (tea and coffee

.Refrain from smoking and stay away from the places where smoking

.Drink 2-3 liters of water, equivalent to at least 8-10 cups per day

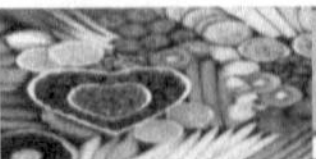

Dietary guidelines for a nursing mother:

.Reducing stimulant drinks such as tea and coffee

Avoid marinated and fried foods and foods with strong odors
.such as onions and garlic, as they affect the taste of milk

Eat a balanced diet that includes all food combinations of
.meat, milk, vegetables, fruits and starches

.Drink enough fluids in general and milk in particular

.Take iron tablets

.Avoid physical and mental stress and agitation

Drink 2-3 liters of water, equivalent to 8-10 cups per day, at
.least

Breastfeeding:

It is the process of supplying the baby with the mother's milk
by placing the child on the mother's chest immediately after
birth, or during the first hour after birth.

Mother's milk consists in the first days of the birth of her baby
from the yellow matter (colostrum milk), which is excreted
immediately after birth. Mother's milk contains all the
nutrients necessary and sufficient for the child's mental and
physical development, and also contains immunomodulators
and antibodies that help protect the child from diseases.

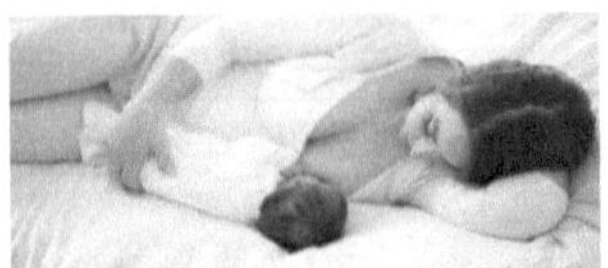

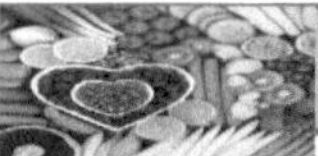

All nutrients in milk are very similar to all mothers, especially that mother who strives to eat a healthy balanced food, but the amount of fatty substances in breast milk varies from time to time during the day, at the end of the day it is higher than at the beginning, and the amount in The milk of the last infant is higher than at the beginning of the infant, and the shorter the period between the infant and the infant, the greater the amount of fat in the mother's milk.

Then breastfeeding should be on demand, i.e. breastfeeding the child at the time that the child wants or the mother needs, without restrictions on the duration or number of feeding times, and this helps to meet the needs of the child when he is hungry, or the needs of the mother when her breasts are full, and that is by keeping the mother and the child together During the day and at night, placing the child on the breast when he shows signs of hunger, such as putting his hand in his mouth, or searching for his mouth for the breast, or other movements, and may eventually resort to crying.

Breastfeeding is a daily conversation between a mother and her baby, not just a transfer of nutrients and vitamins, but rather a transmission of feelings, feelings, and thoughts.

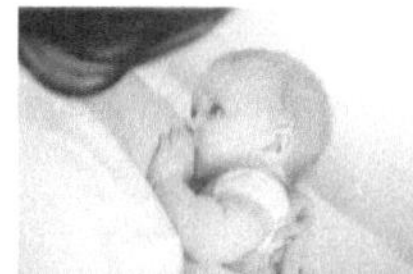

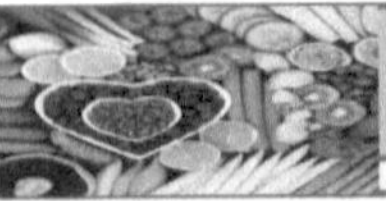

Benefits of breastfeeding:

Benefits of breastfeeding the child:

Providing an adequate and complete food for the child .1

Providing clean, unpolluted food, as it passes directly from .2
the mother's breasts into the child's mouth, thereby not
exposed to contamination

Helping the growth of the jaw and teeth properly .3

Providing food that protects the child by strengthening the .4
immune system, and thus reducing the risk of developing
several diseases.

Benefits of breastfeeding the mother:

.It helps in causing uterine contractions, which reduces blood
loss and stops bleeding and helps restore the size of the uterus
to what it was before pregnancz

.Help the mother to regain her pre-pregnancy weight

.Reduces the risk of pre-menopausal breast and ovarian cancer

.Reduces the occurrence of postpartum depression

.The relationship and the emotional bond between the mother
and the child are strengthened

.It provides the mother with the comfort and time to care for
her baby and family and makes feeding the child a comfortable
night

.Delays the occurrence of a new pregnancy, especially in the
first six months after birth if the breastfeeding is pure

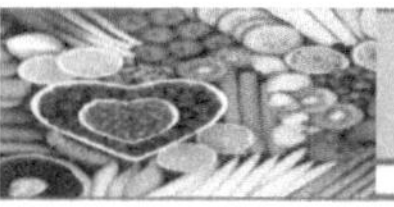

Exclusive breastfeeding:

It is the total dependence on breastfeeding during the first six months after birth and not giving the child water or other fluids or any foods, i.e. that the child's nutrition is limited to the mother's milk only during the first six months of his life, and the World Health Organization and UNICEF recommended that the child be given breast milk Only during the first six months of his life, because the mother's milk meets the needs of the child without any additives, and it is advised to add complementary foods when the child reaches the six months while continuing to breastfeed.

Early breastfeeding immediately after birth:

It means giving the infant the opportunity to breastfeed from his mother as soon as possible after birth, and to stay with his mother in her room the entire time after birth.

How to breastfeed my child ??

The child must be given the opportunity to breastfeed his mother's breastfeeding completely during the first six months after birth, and not to be given water, or other fluids, or any supplementary foods, and when the child reaches six months, it must start adding complementary foods while continuing to breastfeed the child until He is two years old.

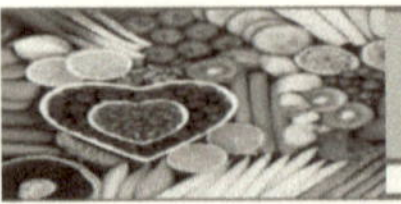

It is imperative for the mother to breastfeed her baby in a proper and correct way, and for breastfeeding to be comfortable in both parties, ideally, the following is recommended:

.Take into account that the position of the mother is comfortable, whether sitting or lying down to breastfeed her baby

.The mother attaches her baby to her chest and the infant's body is adjacent to her body, and his upper ear, shoulder and upper pelvis are on one straightness

.With her forearm the mother rested the child's seat in addition to his head and shoulders

.The mother supports the breasts with her other hand, and brings it closer to the baby's mouth (all the breasts come close to the baby's mouth, not just the nipple)

.The child is well positioned on the breast so that his chin is in contact with the breast (at the lower end of the aura) and his upper lip is opposite to the nipple, making the mother the nipple touching the upper lip of the child (and urges the child to open his mouth)

.The mother waits for the child to open his mouth wide, pulling his head toward the nipple so that the lower lip is inverted, touching the lower end of the aura, and the child grabs the breast properly

.The protrusion formed by the nipple and most areola fills the child's mouth

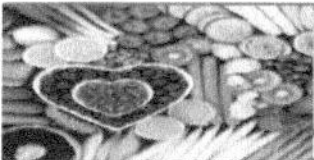

The child should be allowed to finish breastfeeding the first breast before the second is presented to him, and some children may be satisfied with one breast

It is preferable for the mother to breastfeed the child during the night, because during this period the prolactin hormone that stimulates milk production is stimulated.

Breastfeeding working mother:

The working mother is to maintain breastfeeding the milk squeezing method, which is an effective way to give the child the pain of milk during work. The following is an explanation of how milk is squeezed:

There are two ways to squeeze milk:

1 Hurricane by hand:

.Easy, quick and inexpensive operation, and it is considered the cleanest and best way to get breast milk. It takes no more than 20-30 minutes

.Find a quiet and private place

.Wash hands thoroughly with soap and water

.Prepare a clean cup with a tight lid with a wide opening and pour boiling water into it, then the mother will empty boiling water directly from the bowl before the start of the hurricane process

.Place the hand on the aura of the breast so that the thumb and index finger are facing on the outside of the aura

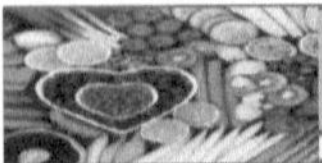

Pressing the breast back toward the chest with the thumb and forefinger, bearing in mind that the mother does not move her fingers over the breast

.Bring the thumb and forefinger together to milk, then relax the hand and press again

.Repeat the same process by moving the two fingers to another place around the areola

.Then the mother stores the squeezed milk where she can leave it at room temperature for a period ranging between 4-6 hours, or in the refrigerator for up to 48 hours provided that it is not placed in the refrigerator door, and it can also be kept in the freezer for two weeks

2 Hurricane aspirator:

The hood should be easy to use, comfortable, effective and harmless to the mother and all parts of the hood can be easily cleaned

The risks of artificial feeding on a child:

.Increased risk of diarrhea

.Exposure to acute respiratory diseases

.Infection as a result of contamination of synthetic milk while preparing it

.The risk of a deficiency in some nutrients

.Child exposure to chronic diseases and some types of cancer

.Increased incidence of infection with diseases of the digestive system and ear infections

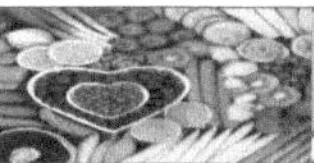

Complementary foods and breastfeeding:

The child needs complementary foods in addition to breast milk when he is completing his sixth month, as he gradually gets used to eating other foods.

Supplementary foods are prepared especially for the child, or it is from the family's usual eating after the child has completed his first year but after mashing or cutting it or adding other types to provide nutrients in the food.

Basic rules for introducing complementary foods:

In order for the mother to ensure that the foods she provides to her child are sufficient and rich in the nutrients it needs, she must observe the following rules when starting to provide complementary foods for the child:

. Begin introducing complementary foods at the age of 6 months and continue breastfeeding for two years and more

. Serving one kind of pureed food every time and adding a new kind of food every 3 days

. Diversification of foods provided to ensure the availability of nutrients: meat, chicken, fish or eggs, milk products that are a good source of calcium, vegetables and fruits rich in vitamins, or foods that contain fatty substances being an important and main source of energy and try to reduce juices, and avoid tea or coffee Or any sweetened liquids or any soft drinks that contain soda

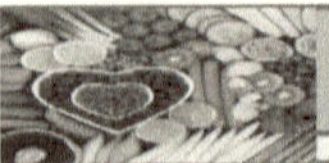

. Begin in small quantities with gradually increasing it as the child grows

. Provide a class of food to avoid allergies

. Serve soft and soft food first, then gradually increase its texture

. Use a cup or spoon, and do not use the feeding bottle

. The food provided must be fresh, clean and well cooked. If it is not placed in the refrigerator, it should be served to the child within two hours of preparing it

. Avoid adding sugar, salt, or spices to the child's food

. Ensure the child is nourished during his illness and increase the number of complementary meals after recovery while continuing to breastfeed

. Encourage the child to eat complementary foods and sit with him, and not be forced to eat, but the time of the meal should be sufficient, joyful and amusing

. It is recommended to give it water and liquid after finishing the meal, not during it

. Take care to wash vegetables and fruits thoroughly before preparing them, as well as wash the baby's hands before feeding him

Note:

The best food to start with in complementary foods is ground rice

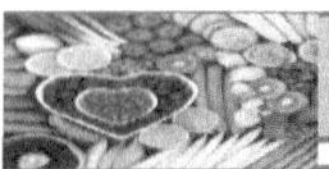

Food of the seventh month:

The main purpose during this month is to get used to eating foods as well as breastfeeding with a spoon and a cup.

Number of meals	Quantity	Meals menu
Feeding on request + 2 meals from the meal menu	Mother's milk	
	1-2 tbsp	Ground rice (boiled
	Half a medium apple Two-thirds of medium sized bananas	Mashed Apple ((Fresh and Boiled Pureed Banana ((fresh and boiled
	1-2 tbsp	Mashed potatoes ((fresh and boiled Mashed carrots ((fresh and boiled
This list provides the child with 100 calories		

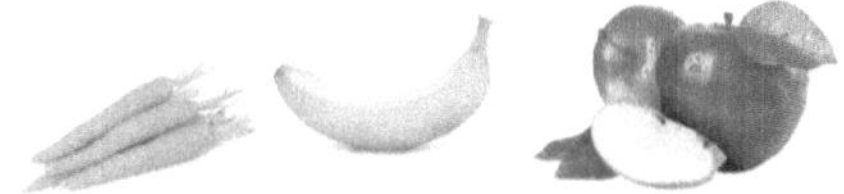

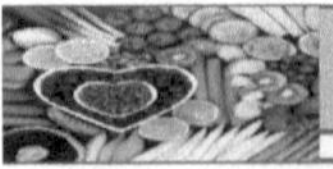

Food for the eighth and ninth months:

During this period, the child's needs for energy, building and growth foods increase, and in the ninth month, the mother begins encouraging the child to hold food.

Number of meals	Quantity	Meals menu
Feeding on request + three meals from the meal menu	Mother's milk	
	2-3 tbsp A small slice of bread	Boiled rice, boiled lentils, peeled beans, bread
	Half a grain of medium size fruit 100 ml of juice, about a quarter of a small cup	Boiled and mashed fruit, one kind of fruit juice
	2-3 tbsp tablespoon of broth	Mixture of boiled vegetables with chicken or meat broth
	Tablespoon Tablespoon One egg	Boiled chicken pieces very small Mashed chicken liver Boiled egg yolk
This list provides the child with 200 calories		

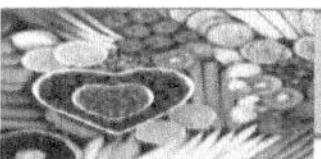

Food for the 10-12 months:

During this period, the child's needs for energy, building and growth foods increase, and it is noted that dairy products can be started.

Number of meals	Quantity	Meals menu
Feeding on request	Mother's milk	
+ three meals from the meal menu + snack	tablespoons 2-3 Medium slice of bread tablespoons 2-3 tablespoons 2-3	Boiled rice, pasta, boiled lentils, peeled beans, bread, rice with milk, pudding ((milk, orange
	Half a grain of medium size fruit 200 ml of juice, about half a small cup	Boiled and mashed fruit One kind fruit juice
	1-4 tbsp 2 tbsp broth	Mixture of boiled vegetables with chicken or meat broth
	2 tbsp 2 tbsp 2 tbsp One egg Two slices Half a cup	Boiled chicken pieces very small Mashed chicken liver Grilled or boiled fish Boiled egg yolk White cheese Yogurt
This list provides the child with 300-400 calories		

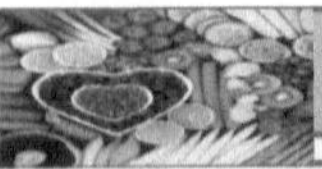

Food for the 12-24 months:

The child begins eating family food, and the child can also be given honey, cake and biscuits.

Number of meals	Quantity	Meals menu
Feeding on demand + three meals from the meal menu + two snacks	Mother's milk	
	2-3 tbsp A medium sized slice of bread 3 tbsp 3 tbsp	Boiled rice, pasta, boiled lentils, peeled beans, bread, rice with milk, pudding ((milk, orange
	One medium sized fruit 400 ml of juice, or about a small cup	Boiled or fresh fruit depending on softness One kind fruit juice
	4 tbsp 2 tbsp	Mixture of boiled vegetables with chicken or meat broth
	3 tbsp 3 tbsp 3 tbsp 3 tbsp One egg 3 slices Cup	Boiled chicken pieces very small Mashed chicken liver Grilled or boiled fish Boiled or minced red meat Boiled eggs White cheese Yogurt
This list provides the child with 500-600 calories		

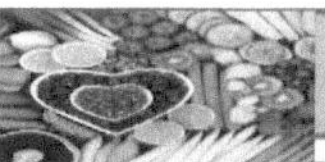

Improve adolescent nutrition:

Adolescent nutrition can be improved through several measures:

. Eat enough and adequate food at specific times and follow healthy eating habits

. Avoid excessive eating of foods, especially those rich in sugar and fat content

. Reducing the intake of sweets, fast food, and soft drinks

. Do physical exercise regularly to burn extra calories and strengthen muscles

. Make sure to eat breakfast in the morning

. Ensure that poultry and derivatives and other meats are cooked, and that the tools and places for cutting meat are cleaned to prevent germs, and that food that is purchased by street vendors should not be eaten. Food should be preserved in a healthy way and wash vegetables and fruits with water before using them, eating pasteurized milk

. Eat a balanced diet of various food groups

. Control of infection with parasites that can be transmitted by food, drink, etc

. Combating a lack of environmental needs (such as iodine, fluoride and iron deficiency) by taking nutritional supplements

. Provide clean water and ensure food safety

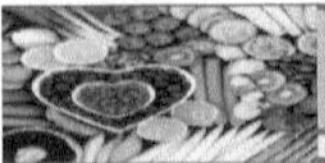

Personal hygiene is the set of habits and practices that a person does to preserve his health and smell, it is considered the pillar of health and an important factor in respecting people and the source of vitality and activity for the human being, so attention must be paid to personal hygiene.

Your guide to personal hygiene in simple points:

1 Body odor:

. You should wear clean outerwear, and change your underwear daily especially in the summer

. Change clothes dirty or sweaty as soon as possible

. The case should be washed daily after wearing it

. The watch and jewelry should be removed during work to prevent carrying dust and germs

. The shoe should be cleaned when entering the home

2 Bathing:

. Daily in all seasons every morning, or at least three times a week and after every sporting activity

. Make sure to use a clean and dry towel, wash it regularly and not share it with the rest of the family

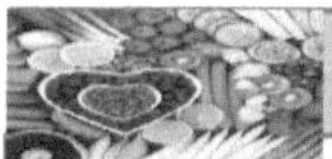

3 Hair:

. Wash especially long hair, at least every two days

. Regularly cut or damage damaged hair

. In the event of scabs or lice, a dermatologist should be consulted

4 The ear:

. Regular cleaning around and outside the ear with the finger while taking a shower

. Clean the ears of wax material carefully and without exaggeration

5 Get rid of bad breath:

. Drink more water

. Brushing and brushing teeth

. Stay away from tobacco products

6 Nails:

. Trim nails weekly

. Wash nails thoroughly with soap and water daily

7 Legs:

. Foot wash regularly, especially between toes

. Not wearing tight shoes

. It is not preferable to wear the same shoes for as long as possible

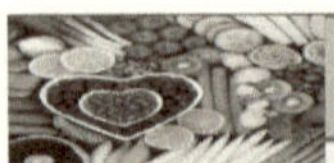

House cleanliness:

Cleanliness of the house is an essential part of the mental and physical health of its members, and a reflection of their image and lifestyle. Each family needs to put in place a system to maintain the cleanliness of the home, including all its details, and involving all family members.

The kitchen:

. Set aside a specific bowl for dishwashing, in which you place clean water, dishwashing sponge and sponge, and do not use the kitchen sponge for any other uses such as cleaning the bathroom, floor or dust

. Replace the kitchen sponge every two weeks, as the used sponge contains many germs and bacteria and it is difficult to completely disinfect it

. Clean the sinks and the surfaces you use to prepare food and dry them well, immediately after each use

. Use disposable paper towels, when cleaning very dirty or contaminated items, or when handling raw foods to avoid the transfer of bacteria to other tools or foods

. Wipe the dining table with soap and water after eating

. Clean the gas with water and soap after each use and do not leave food traces to accumulate on it

. Create a kitchen trash can and lid appropriate to its size, and do not throw any waste into it before placing a bag inside

. Put food and waste scrap in the trash can in the kitchen, and dispose of it on a daily basis

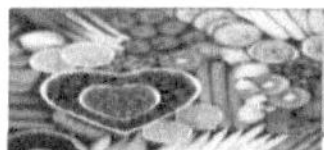

. Open the windows daily and in all seasons, for at least two hours, to allow air and sun to enter the rooms

. Change the bed sheets and wash the bed sheets at a high temperature once a week, as needed

. Do not put food or eat in the bedrooms to avoid insects

. Wipe floors with water and detergent at least three times a week and when needed, with the goal of removing visible dirt

The toilet:

. Clean the surface and interior of the toilet and the sink daily, and make sure to permanently envelop the toilet cover before pressing the water flush, to prevent the spread of germs

. Clean the water drains every three months with a medicine that eliminates lime with boiling water, not leaving dirt or hair to accumulate

. Cleanse the toilet immediately after using it by a sick person suffering from infections or diarrhea

. Ventilate the bathroom by opening the windows

Clothing:

Separate the clothes when washing them so that no bacteria .transfer between clothes

Wash the underwear at high temperatures to sterilize it from .microbes and germs